A Paramedic's Guide: Wilderness First Aid

Copyright Lance Hodge, 2014

ISBN 978-1500182663

Printed in the United States of America

A Paramedic's Guide:
Wilderness First Aid

By Lance Hodge, Paramedic

Contents

A Paramedic's Guide:
WILDERNESS FIRST AID

By Lance Hodge, Paramedic

This booklet is intended to provide you with the basic skills and knowledge to treat serious injuries and illnesses in the backcountry, or anywhere, even at home. Many 'Wilderness First Aid' courses devote significant time to the use of environmental materials for first aid care, including many methods that are impractical and unworkable in a real emergency. In this booklet we will limit our discussion to the use of approved materials and methods for quickly and effectively treating injuries and illnesses in remote areas. Our goal is to be prepared to act quickly and appropriately, including the use of your backpack or home first aid kit to offer the needed supplies.

The author has the experience of over 15,000 emergency responses to 9-1-1 calls as a Paramedic in the Los Angeles City Fire Department over the course of 13 years, as well as experience as a Reserve Deputy on the Sheriff's Search & Rescue team, and over 20 years' experience as the primary instructor of a college EMT Program.

The goal is simple; learn to provide the most appropriate first aid treatment for injuries and illnesses until advanced help is available.

Our major concerns are serious lacerations and bleeding, fractures, eye injuries, and allergic reactions. Many remedies are available for miscellaneous complaints such as headache, stomach ache, diarrhea, cough and fever. A brief list of over-the-counter treatments is included, although more serious injuries and illnesses will be our focus. You will discover that most first aid is a combination of common sense and preparedness.

~

The following supplies represent a first aid kit appropriate for backcountry use, with the essentials necessary for most situations you might encounter (excluding medications).

Suggested first aid kit:
(Bandaging materials should be in a sealed bag to avoid contamination)

1 leg splint, 24", plastic, 2 triangular bandages, 4 roller bandages 4",1 rescue scissors, 6 butterfly bandages, large, 6 Band-Aids x-large, 1 eye wash, 6 butterfly bandages medium, 6 Band-Aids regular, 1 splinter forceps, 2 4x4 dressing, 2 ea. Pack, 6 Povidone Iodine swabs, 2" tape, 2 5x9 dressings, 6 Antimicrobial hand wipes.

TOPICS:

Lacerations:

(A tear in the skin) If the wound is deep and the skin layer seems separated, forming an open area, stitches may be required when medical care is available. First aid care involves the following steps:

Control of bleeding: Slight bleeding will coagulate and stop when a dressing is applied. Significant active bleeding must first be controlled with 'direct pressure'. **If the wound is dirty, quickly wash the contaminants away with water**, then:

1. Place a dressing over the wound (4x4 or 5x9) and apply 'firm' constant pressure with your hand. DO NOT RELEASE the pressure for 5 minutes.
2. Use several 4x4 dressings folded to form a firm "lump" the size of the wound, and a roller bandage to hold the dressing to apply a 'pressure dressing'. Pull the bandage snug over the wound but allow less pressure as you wrap around, to avoid creating a tourniquet effect. You want the pressure directly over the firm lump of dressing, not all the way around.
3. If the dressing soaks through, do not remove the blood soaked dressing, apply more dressing material on top of it, and add more pressure.

When bleeding is controlled: (A pressure dressing can be slowly and carefully removed taking care not to break open the wound and cause bleeding, and a more long term dressing can be applied. Use caution not to reopen an arterial wound) Don't remove if you don't have to.

1. Wash the wound carefully with clean water and pat the area dry. (Use extreme care if the wound initially involved serious active bleeding)
2. Use antiseptic swabs to thoroughly 'paint' the wound with antiseptic solution
3. (You may need to shave hair from the area before using this bandage) Use several 'butterfly bandages' to pull together skin that is separated (these serve as 'temporary' stitches that pull the wound back together, decreasing the chance of infection, reducing further damage and drying due to exposed tissue, and allows healing to begin)
4. Cover the area with a clean dressing to avoid contamination.

Fractures: (Sprains, strains, dislocations)
(A fracture may be obvious if broken bones are exposed or in the case of an obvious deformity) With pain, swelling, and loss of movement, we 'suspect' a possible fracture and treat it as if it is. We cannot tell if a part is simply sprained or strained (sometimes a pop or crack will be heard with damage to tendons or ligaments in a sprain or strain). Treat such injuries as if it is a fracture.

Fractures:

1. Immobilize the injured part using a splint. Apply gentle in-line traction as you lift the injury onto the splint. (Enough pull to slightly separate the bone ends) The splint must be snug to prevent movement of the part and must <u>immobilize the joint above and below the injured part</u>. The farther the splint extends past the joint above and below the fracture the more stable it will be.
2. Use roller bandage or tape to secure the splint, for fractures of the lower arm or leg. (If roller bandage is used, tie in bows to allow for removal and readjustment of the splint in the event of other needed care and/or to readjust for swelling).
3. Use a sling and swath for fractures of the shoulder, clavicle, and upper arm.
4. <u>Severely angulated fractures can be realigned to proper position using slight in-line traction</u>. **(Do not try to realign fractures involving a joint area)** splint such fractures in the position you find them, cutting, bending, and taping your splint to fit the fracture.
5. For foot and ankle injuries, it may be necessary to use tape or roller bandage to stabilize the injury instead of a splint, if the person 'must' walk out for medical care.

<u>Eye injury</u>: (Dust, sand, windblown objects, and bugs, account for most eye injuries/irritation) Scratches to the cornea cannot be detected in the field and will

require careful inspection and antibiotic treatment when medical care is available. Our treatment will include:

1. Flush the eye with eyewash solution or water. (The upper and lower eyelids must be lifted up to flush those areas)
2. For continued pain or irritation, the eye can be covered with a light dressing (piece of 4X4 dressing) held lightly by roller bandage (Irritation from a scratched cornea may last for days and feel as if something is still present)

Blisters: Many backpackers have discovered their own blister treatment from trial and error. The use of Moleskin or Band-Aids to reduce shoe contact to the injured area is one common treatment. (Use the adhesive Moleskin on the 'boot' rather than applying to the skin, there is often significant injury to the skin when removing a soiled moleskin!)

Have a second pair of shoes: Comfortable tennis shoes, or flip-flops, are a lifesaver in the event of significant blisters. Your goal is to relieve the pain and reduce continued irritation of the area while keeping the injury as clean as possible to lessen the chance of infection.

DO NOT POP BLISTERS (Sometimes hikers feel they 'must' pop blisters to relieve the pain to allow for continued travel) If you do, use a disinfected pin to relieve the fluid, while leaving the skin intact, then;

If a blister is open:

1. Twice daily application of antiseptic and clean Band-Aid/dressing is recommended.
2. (Allow the area to dry by exposing to the air for several hours each day).
3. Reapply antiseptic and clean Band-Aid/dressing daily.

Splinter:

1. Remove with tweezers
2. Apply antiseptic
3. Cover with Band-Aid
4. Clean the area and reapply antiseptic daily.

Burns: The most common burns will be sunburn (pain and reddening), and possibly second-degree burn (blisters). Prevent sunburn by using a high SPF waterproof sunscreen lotion/spray, and by using clothing and hats to reduce exposure. Benadryl cream may reduce some sunburn pain and swelling. Burns with blisters should be kept clean and allowed to heal. DO NOT pop blisters from burns if possible; this only increases your chance of infection.

If the blister is open: wash with soap and water, apply antiseptic, cover with Band-Aid/dressing, and keep clean. Reapply the antiseptic and a clean Band-Aid/dressing daily.

Allergic reactions: Could be caused from a reaction to food, environmental sources (pollen, grass, etc.) or a reaction to a bite or sting. (Our biggest concern is a 'severe' allergic reaction that might cause trouble with breathing as airways constrict, which may begin with an itchy throat, coughing, hoarseness, slight wheezing, or a feeling of tightness in the chest). Most allergic reactions will be limited to some local swelling, redness, and itching. One of the most effective treatments is Diphenhydramine (Benadryl).

The over-the-counter dose of Benadryl is 25mg per pill. The normal therapeutic dose for significant allergic reaction is 50-75mg. (Such uses of medications should be discussed with your doctor). Treatment for an obvious allergic reaction should include immediate treatment with Benadryl. If the reaction involves trouble breathing, or wheezing, use 50-75mg.

Note: Benadryl is very safe but can cause sleepiness, and can be used as a sleep aid!

(Benadryl cream can be used along with oral medication for application to redness or swelling of affected skin)

Poison Oak: The plant oils can be spread by touching other body parts and may remain on clothing. (Use washcloth with soap and water, avoiding contact with hands). Use Caladryl cream on effected skin. Rash/itching may take up to a week to subside.

Bites & stings: The goal of first aid for bites & stings is to clean the wound and treat symptoms that appear.

If complaints involve redness, swelling, puffiness, or itchiness, see the treatment for Allergic Reactions above.

Bees: The bee may leave its stinger in the skin, and it may have a portion of the bee's abdomen still attached to it. This can be removed with a tweezers, making sure the stinger is grabbed as close as possible to the skin so as not to squeeze the bee tissue that may contain the poison sac.

1. After removing the stinger (if found), wash the area with soap and water.
2. Apply antiseptic swab to the 'immediate' area.
3. Apply Benadryl cream (if available) to area around the sting.
4. Cover with Band-Aid to avoid contamination of area.
5. Treat with oral Benadryl if signs of allergic reaction are present.

Spiders: Black Widow (causing abdominal cramping), and Brown Recluse (causing an area of dead tissue at the bite site, usually many hours after a bite, that may become infected), are the spiders of serious concern. Other spider bites may cause some pain, and in some individuals may result in allergic reaction. (Use Benadryl or Benadryl cream) Wounds should be washed, antiseptic applied, and covered with a Band-Aid.

**Ticks**: Ticks are common in many backcountry areas. They often wait on the ends of plants and attach themselves to you as you brush by. Check your clothing often for ticks. Check your body at the end of the day, especially armpits, groin, and neck.

1. _Wear light-colored clothing in areas known for ticks to better detect them on you._
2. _If a tick is attached to your skin: Grab 'gently' with a tweezers, near its head, and 'slowly' pull until 'it' releases and can be removed. (At this point you want the tick alive, so that 'it' can let go. Otherwise its head or mouthparts might be left in your skin)_
3. _Once the tick is removed: Kill the tick! (Wash your hands if you touched the tick)_
4. _Cleanse the area with soap and water._
5. _Treat the bite area with antiseptic swab._
6. _Cover with a Band-Aid._
7. _Watch the wound for signs of infection, redness, swelling, and seek medical care as soon as available (Several illnesses can be spread by ticks)_

**Snake**: Non-poisonous snakes may bite and cause a bite wound that should be cleaned with soap and water then treated with antiseptic and a dressing.

Rattlesnake: 'Avoid being bitten' by never putting your hands where you cannot see. Shake out boots, blankets, sleeping bags, before using. Watch the trail ahead! Use a **walking stick** in snake country to check the area before you step, they may not rattle before they bite.

If bitten: DO NOT cut the area or try to suck out venom. Cutting and sucking creates a huge risk of infection and is _not_ effective in removing venom. DO NOT apply a tourniquet. Remain calm; most people will not die from a rattlesnake bite. Seek medical care as soon as you can. DO NOT delay medical care. There is no prehospital first aid; you will need medical care and anti-venin at the hospital. TIME is critical, get to help, walk out if you can if rescue will be prolonged.

Misc. other bites or stings:
Wasps, hornets, ants, tarantula, etc., etc.
1.   Wash the area with soap and water.
2.   Apply Benadryl cream to area.
3.   Take Benadryl tablet(s) if signs of allergic reaction.

If distress is mild you might decide to continue your trip, if significant distress or long delay for further care, end your trip and seek proper medical care!

A General overview of some common medical conditions, as well as some treatments and concerns

Illnesses: A list of some typical over-the-counter treatments for various symptoms is available on page 27 of this booklet. (As always, discuss specific medications with your doctor if you have any medical conditions or are taking any medications).

Coughing/trouble breathing: Our major concern with persistent coughing in the wilderness, especially at higher altitudes, is that it could signal the onset of pulmonary edema (fluid in the lungs) known as **Altitude Sickness**. This is most often caused by a sudden change in altitude (usually at altitudes over 10,000 ft.), and can progress to a life-threatening condition. If pulmonary edema is suspected you <u>must</u> get the person to a lower altitude right away, THAT is the only **cure** you will have.

Signs of pulmonary edema include: Coughing, trouble catching their breath, difficulty speaking, blueness around the lips, and the sound of lung fluid (gurgling, bubbling, crackling) when breathing and/or coughing.

Other coughing: Respiratory problems can result from many things including, irritation from dust, dry air, overly moist air, and illness. Other than rest, and decreasing the stress by relieving the person of some of the weight in their pack, we can only hope the illness is short-lived. Obviously a person in significant distress should leave the backcountry and seek medical care.

Wheezing: A narrowing of air passages may cause wheezing (a whistling sound on breathing in, or out, or both). This can be a sign of someone experiencing an asthma attack (those with asthma 'should' have appropriate medication available to treat wheezing). Those who do not have asthma may experience wheezing accompanied by shortness of breath due to the stress of exercise, allergic reactions, and changing or unfamiliar environmental conditions bringing about irritation to the airways and lungs. Any sign of respiratory distress should not be ignored; the person should stop physical activity until the wheezing stops; since wheezing could be the result of an allergic reaction, taking Benadryl may be advised.

Headache: Headache, even severe and recurrent, is not uncommon in the backcountry. Changes in altitude and the stresses of exertion can cause them, along with lack of food or changes in diet, and dehydration. (Make sure you drink 'plenty' of water!)

Aspirin can be taken as a precaution and may help prevent headaches from occurring. There could be some correlation in the blood thinning effects of aspirin in preventing headaches. ('Aspirin' has this beneficial effect, <u>not</u> Tylenol, Ibuprofen, etc.)

1. *Take a single low-dose (81mg) Aspirin tablet in the morning and again in the evening. Since a regular aspirin tablet contains 325mg. you can safely take several more low-dose Aspirin if a headache continues. (See your doctor before taking any medication to make sure it is safe for 'you').*
2. *Make sure you are eating appropriately and drinking* **plenty** *of water in the backcountry.*
3. *Take more frequent rest stops and drink more frequently if headaches persist.*

<u>**Dizziness**</u>: *The most common causes of dizziness when hiking is a combination of exertion, altitude, dehydration, and lower food intake (loss of calories). Take care to eat and drink properly, physically condition 'before' entering the backcountry, and take time to acclimatize to higher altitudes, if possible, by spending a day or two at the higher altitude before heading out, or by planning a slower ascension to higher altitudes.*

Fainting: Fainting is usually a sign of over-exertion, and inadequate water or food intake. Fainting 'can' be a sign of serious medical problems.

'After' a person has fainted:

1. Lay them **flat** on their back with their feet elevated about 12-18" (Shock position) As long as they are breathing adequately **do not rush to wake them or to sit them up**. Do not raise their head, keep it flat. It may take a minute or so to recover. 'Incontinence' (loss of bladder control) is common after fainting. Sometimes a very short 'seizure' will precede fainting (due to lack of blood circulating to the brain). If the fainting spell was due to one of the simple causes listed the person should recover shortly. **Don't** sit them up right away.
2. Check for signs of injury if they fell.

Seizure: Seizures are caused by a disruption of blood supply to the brain or a disturbance in the normal electrical activity in the brain. Someone with 'epilepsy' will occasionally have seizures and is probably on medication to help control them. Expect full body shaking, clenching of the jaw, stiffening and shaking of the arms and legs. Their face may turn bluish from temporary lack of oxygen, and their eyes may roll up in their head. A person who is epileptic will most likely have a short seizure (30 seconds to one minute) followed by a period of sleepiness or confusion. (Do not rush to awaken them. This sleepy period could be short or last for 20-30 minutes). For people who do not have epilepsy and experience a first-time seizure we suspect several possibilities: Stroke, brain tumor, drug overdose or reaction, or severe lack of oxygen, low blood sugar from poor diet, severe dehydration, or fever (A slight seizing activity can precede a fainting episode)

1. Move objects out of the way so that they are not hitting things as they shake, do NOT hold them or try to stop the shaking.
2. DO NOT put <u>anything</u> in their mouth, they cannot 'swallow' their tongue, and if they are going to bite it, it cannot be prevented safely since their jaw is usually clenched. A tongue injury, if it occurs, may be ugly but is usually minor.
3. Let them lie down to recover. They may be combative due to a temporary lack of oxygen to the brain. (Do not try to arouse them, let them sleep. This sleepy period should last less than 30 minutes)
4. When they begin to regain consciousness have them continue to lie down for some time to 'fully' recover before sitting or standing up.

<u>Nosebleed</u>: (Often the result of dry air, exertion, and/or altitude) DO NOT SWALLOW

BLOOD (this may cause stomach irritation and vomiting). If the bleeding is minor dripping DO NOT pinch the nose. Just sit or lie down, head raised, and relax, it should stop on its own. (<u>Do not swallow blood & Do not blow your nose, spit out blood</u>).

Nosebleed with 'significant' bleeding:

1. Sit down. Lean forward 'slightly' (DO NOT lower the head between the legs, which causes extra pressure and increased bleeding)
2. Spit out any blood that drips into the back of the throat.
3. Pinch the upper part of the nose 'firmly' as close to the head as possible.
   <u>Continue</u> pinching for 'at least' 5 minutes 'without' letting go. (DO NOT blow your nose after bleeding is controlled)

Stomach ache: Some over-the-counter remedies will help with stomach ache, which is usually brought on by changes in foods and over-exertion. On a long trip, of a week or more, you could develop stomach ache due to intestinal parasites from non-filtered water. This will require medical treatment when you return to civilization, and may be accompanied by diarrhea.

Nausea/vomiting: A common occurrence on the first day or two of a backcountry trip, especially when unaccustomed to the altitude and physical stresses.

1. Benadryl is also an anti-emetic, which can reduce the possibility of vomiting.
2. Make sure fluids continue to be consumed, but try small, frequent sips.

Cramps: Can be caused by too much physical activity, which over taxes the muscles and deprives the tissue of needed fluid or minerals. (Also, see 'Giardia' under Diarrhea)

1. Make sure water intake is sufficient.
2. Drink 'electrolyte' solutions such as 'Gatorade' or 'Power aid'.

Diarrhea: Our worry here would be 'Giardia' (a protozoal parasite water contaminant) that will require medication to eliminate. (It will probably take a week or more for Giardia symptoms to occur) There are some over-the-counter diarrhea medications that will help to relieve some symptoms. Sometimes simple diarrhea is brought about by changes in diet and should resolve shortly.

Fever: Fever is a sign of infection (Ranging from a simple cold to a serious infection requiring medication and medical care). Fever reducing medications can relieve some symptoms and lower the fever, but treatment should be sought as soon as possible.

Stroke: Caused by a rupture of a vessel or a blocked vessel in the brain. Results in one-sided paralysis, slurred speech. This person needs prompt medical treatment. Keep their head somewhat elevated if possible.

Heart Attack: Chest pain or 'pressure', pain to the arm or jaw, nausea, vomiting, pale, cool, sweaty skin, irregular pulse. This is a serious life-threatening situation. The person should be kept calm, lay flat with feet raised 12-18", do not let them further exert themselves if possible. Although possible, heart attack is rare in younger people with no medical problems. (If there is pain on breathing it is most likely a lung related problem, not a heart attack). Rest before continuing.

> * **Aspirin**: Taken immediately for a heart attack can reduce the severity of a heart attack. **Dose**: (2) 325mg. tablets (which equals (8) low-dose 81mg. tablets.

Appendicitis: Severe right lower abdominal pain and tenderness. May also be accompanied by loss of appetite and fever. Patient needs prompt medical care.

Choking: (See the CPR/FBAO, Foreign Body Airway Obstruction, guide at the back of this booklet)

Note regarding 'severe trauma', unable to continue, and death: (See CPR guide at back of this booklet… but remember that CPR is only useful if advanced medical care, and defibrillation, will be available soon, within about 15-20 minutes. Beyond a relatively short time it will become impossible to resuscitate due to brain damage and metabolic deterioration). If CPR fails to revive the person in 15-20 minutes, and it will be 'hours' before help, continued resuscitation efforts are most likely futile.

Pre-cordial thump: In the absence of access to defibrillation or advanced medical care, you can attempt a pre-cordial thump **only** on a non-breathing, pulseless, unresponsive person, which 'may' in some cases stop ventricular fibrillation and allow a heartbeat to return.

1. Hold your fist 12" above the person's chest.
2. Deliver a **very** firm, rapid blow to the middle of the breastbone (between the nipples).
3. Check the carotid pulse in the neck for a pulse, for at least 10 seconds.
4. If no pulse, repeat the pre-cordial thump.
5. Check the pulse in the neck for at least 10 seconds after each blow.
6. If no pulse after four or five attempts, and no medical care is near, resuscitation is most likely futile.

Death:
If a death occurs while in the backcountry, the person should be left in a tent if possible, to decrease the likelihood of predation by animals, while others go for help.

<u>**Unable to continue/left behind**</u>:
In the event of a severe injury or someone unable to continue, someone should stay with the injured/ill person while others go for help. If someone must be left alone they should be left in a tent in a shaded area, be placed on their side if unconscious, and if conscious have sufficient food, water, and supplies nearby.

<u>**Signs of severe head trauma**</u>: After a fall or blow to the head, if the person is unconscious, you may see signs that indicate significant brain injury such as:

1. One pupil is significantly larger than the other and not reactive to light; a sign of bleeding of and pressure in the brain.
2. Abnormal breathing pattern; extremely deep in and out breaths, or breaths that increase then decrease with long pauses; a sign of pressure on the brain due to bleeding.
3. Clear fluid from the nose or ears can indicate cerebral spinal fluid leakage, which is the sign of a skull fracture.
4. **Posturing**, a stiffening of the body in which the arms and legs stiffen, and arms may bend inward toward the chest or stiffen to the person's side. This is a sign of severe injury to the brain.

Such persons need immediate medical care and surgery. The prognosis is very poor for such a severe injury while in the backcountry.

1. Keep the person warm
2. DO NOT twist their neck or body in case of a hidden injury to the spinal column; keep them straight if you move them.
3. Lay them with their body straight but their head pointed somewhat uphill to relieve some of the pressure to the brain.

Quick general assessment: To check for injury, remove clothing (cut off if necessary to avoid manipulating injured areas).

1. _Look and feel for wounds and deformity_. (Firmly feel and gently move bones and joints checking for instability that may indicate a fracture)
2. _Pupils_: Should be equal size and react to light (shade the eye and remove the shade quickly to watch for reaction to light) One large, non-reactive pupil is a sign of serious head injury (person will most likely be unconscious or extremely disoriented)
3. _Ears and nose_: Clear fluid draining from the ears or nose after head injury and unconsciousness may indicate leaking cerebral spinal fluid, and a skull fracture.

4. _Lungs_: Place ear to chest. Each side should be equal with no noisy breathing.
5. _Abdomen_: Rigidity, swelling, or tenderness could indicate internal bleeding.
6. _Pelvis_: Squeeze firmly the sides of pelvis. Pain or instability could indicate pelvic fracture.
7. _Legs_: Thigh. Swelling and/or deformity could be a sign of a fractured femur.
    > _Fractured hip_: Leg on injured side is shortened and rotated outward.
    > _Dislocated hip_: Injured leg has knee bent and is rotated inward.

Any of these significant findings upon physical exam are signs of potentially serious injury and need prompt medical attention.

**Shock**: Pale, cool, sweaty skin and a rapid pulse are signs of shock (inadequate circulation of blood to vital organs).
1. Lay the person flat, (shock position) raise the legs 12-18". Give fluids if possible. Keep them warm.

*Never force liquids and cause choking, give small sips.

NOTE: There are of course numerous other medical conditions that could be encountered. Specific treatments for medical conditions may vary between individuals. Being prepared for the most common possibilities will help you better prepare for the unexpected. Use your best judgment, and these guidelines, to care for whatever illness or injury you might encounter. Always bring any prescription medications you 'might' need along on your backcountry trip, plan for water sources (always filter or disinfect water), know your route (have an accurate map and a compass), and prepare for inclement weather. Make sure your first aid kit is handy, and make sure 'everyone' in your group knows where it is. Having a few more supplies is better than not enough.

*There are many first-aid books at your local bookstore that give more background information on many of these conditions. Be as knowledgeable as possible, always have a fully stocked first-aid kit and misc. medications that might be useful. **Always filter or chemically treat any backcountry water before using in food or drinking**, and <u>try to avoid risk-taking in the backcountry</u>.*

The following list contains 'some' common over-the-counter medications and their uses:

*Benadryl/Benadryl Cream (Diphenhydramine): *Allergic reaction. The oral medication also serves as an anti-vomiting treatment and as a sleep aid*
Caladryl: *Itching from allergic reaction, poison oak*
Neosporin + Pain relief: *Antibiotic, wound care*
Pepsid AC: *Acid indigestion*
Kaopectate: *Diarrhea & cramping*
*Pepto-Bismol: *Nausea, diarrhea, stomach ache*
*Aspirin: *Pain, fever*
Robitussin 'Flu': *Headache, fever, sneeze, cough, nasal congestion, runny nose*
TheraFlu: *Headache, fever, sneeze, cough, nasal congestion, runny nose*
Gatoraid/Poweraid powdered drink mix: *To replace lost minerals and salts from dehydration.*

* A 'must have' for backcountry travel

Proper planning of backcountry adventures will:

Help insure you know where you're going...

Insure you have the right equipment and supplies...

Instill confidence that you know how to handle unexpected emergencies...

Survival First-aid kits for trauma

• **Misc. supplies**: *1 leg splint, 24", plastic, 1 rescue scissors, 1 eye wash, 1 splinter forceps, 2" tape*

• **Bandage supplies**: *(In sealed bag) 2 triangular bandages, 4 roller bandages, 4", (2) 4x4 dressing, 2 ea. pk., (2) 5x9 dressings, 6 butterfly bandages, large, 6 butterfly bandages, medium, 6 Band-Aids, x-large, 6 Band-Aids, regular, 6 Povidone Iodine swabs, 6 Antimicrobial hand wipes.*

*Always bring a basic survival first aid kit when traveling in the wilderness, and **practice** bandaging and splinting.*

Note: Of course improvised splints, using sticks, will work, but often require some practice and are often not as secure as a manufactured splint. The first aid kit above is quite small and light, and you *could* eliminate the splint, although it can be slipped into a standard backpack taking up almost no extra room.

Critical Emergency Response Training
(C.E.R.T)

The first section was a more immediate and simplified approach to Wilderness First Aid, this section takes a more clinical approach, perhaps best for those with some level of previous training.

Regardless of your experience or previous training, you should find some additional information here, and perhaps some techniques that could be helpful.

What is an emergency?

Quick recognition of true emergencies leads to timely and lifesaving intervention

An Emergency is generally: A situation requiring a rapid response.

In many cases emergencies will involve situations in which your rapid and appropriate response may reduce the chance of further injury, slow the progress of an acute illness, and even lessen property damage. Of course our primary goal is always the protection of persons, the patient and bystanders.

In the pages that follow we will examine some simple treatments for various medical emergencies. Rapid access to the 9-1-1 EMS system is always a priority!

Although much of our first aid is simple, we should not underestimate your ability to provide lifesaving intervention. The first responder or EMT provides 'Most' prehospital lifesaving care through basic life support and first aid, not with advanced equipment or medications.

Safety FIRST! Later we will discuss CPR, initial patient assessments and the A, B, C's of first aid. But perhaps the most important aspect of first aid is 'Safety'. Your PRIMARY concern is YOUR safety. You can't help anyone if you become another patient!

Even before you approach an emergency scene you must ask yourself if it is safe to do so. SLOW DOWN, look at the 'whole' scene, try to look for possible hidden hazards, and do not approach if you believe a danger to you exists. At this point your most valuable action may be in staying back, calling for appropriate help, and keeping others from entering the area.

Hidden Dangers:
•   Falling or loose objects above

- Electrical wiring
- Flammable and/or hazardous materials
- Exposure to disease
- For fights, disputes, or injuries, where is the person responsible?

The initial patient exam

For lack of a better description we will refer to the ill or injured person as your 'patient'.

1. **Shout and Tap**: You have decided it was safe to approach the patient. Now you must determine responsiveness. First look at the person's hands for objects or weapons (leave the scene or remove them if safe to do so.) First shout, "Are you O.K.!" Then 'Firmly' tap the shoulder several times and shout again, "Are you O.K!"

2. **A, B, C's**: (Airway-Breathing-Circulation)

Airway: If the person appears to be breathing (the chest rising and falling), then do not tilt the head back. If you are not able to tell if they are breathing you must attempt to breathe for them (using an airway barrier device for protection). If breaths do not go in, you can then tilt the head using the 'Head-Tilt, Chin-Lift' maneuver. (If breaths do not go in (the chest does not rise) after the second attempt, consider airway obstruction procedures). Later we will discuss neck injury and the airway.

Breathing: Normal breathing is about 12 times a minute. If the person's breathing is significantly less than this, you must 'assist' their breathing so that they receive at least one breath every 5 seconds. (Child and Infant: give one breath every 3 seconds). Give two slow breaths, each one just until the chest rises. (Over inflating the lungs may cause air to enter the stomach that may cause vomiting).

Circulation: (Pulse). This is checked at the neck (Carotid Artery) in adults and children, and the arm, under the bicep muscle (Brachial Artery) in infants. If there 'is' a pulse, monitor the patient's breathing and assist it if necessary, and place the patient in 'recovery position' (on their side) to protect the airway from possible vomiting. If there is no pulse you must begin 'chest compressions' and CPR.

Cardio-Pulmonary Resuscitation: (CPR)

CPR is most effective when begun immediately after the heart stops pumping. Within 4-6 minutes the patient may have suffered from permanent brain injury. The person in cardiac arrest must have access to a 'defibrillator' as quickly as possible for the greatest chance of survival. You must call for Advanced Life Support (ALS) providers (Paramedics) as soon as you realize your patient is in any 'serious' condition such as unconsciousness, trouble breathing, signs of shock (pale, cool, sweaty), altered level of consciousness (confused), etc.

Manikin practice: You should practice CPR compressions and 'breathing' on training manikins. Although you may practice 'mouth-to-mouth' breathing methods, it is assumed that you will have some 'barrier device' during an actual emergency to avoid direct contact with the patient's mouth and/or bodily fluids.

'Standard Precautions' or Body Substance Isolation, BSI; also known as Universal Precautions, is the concept that you treat 'every' person you encounter as if they were infectious, and use barriers (barrier/bag-valve-mask to ventilate, gloves, goggles, gown) to prevent contact with any bodily fluids.

Adult:
(An adult, for CPR purposes, is anyone who has reached puberty). The chest is compressed with the heel of one hand on the lower half of the sternum (breast bone), basically lining up the middle of the heel of the hand with the person's imaginary 'nipple line' with the other hand on top of the first. The chest is compressed 'at least two inches' in depth, at a rate of 100-120 per minute. Two breaths are given after every 30 compressions. (30:2)

Two-person CPR is the same, with one rescuer handling the ventilations and the other doing the chest compressions.

Child:
(From 1-year-old to puberty). The chest is compressed using the heel of only one hand, or two, on the lower half of the sternum. (One or two hands on chest depending on size of child and how much force is needed.) Compressions are two inches deep, at a rate of 100-120 per minute. Two

breath are given after every 30 compressions. (30:2) Note: For children and infants with two rescuers, use 15 compressions and two breaths (15:2)

Infant:
(Newborn to 1-year-old). The chest is compressed using the index and middle finger, placed just below the 'nipple line', at a depth of one and a half inches deep. The rate is 100-120 per minute. Two breaths are given after every 30 compressions. (30:2) Note: For children and infants with two rescuers, use 15 compressions and two breaths (15:2)

First Aid:

First Aid is any care that you give to someone in distress following illness or injury. Your interventions will be simple for the most part but may be critical in the care of the patient. The 'wrong' intervention could result in serious injury or even death to the patient.

Always remember to avoid any action that could result in further injury or complicate the patient's situation.

Sometimes the best action is to call for appropriate help, calm the patient, and take control of the scene, rather than attempt some treatment that could cause more damage to the patient.

Medical vs. Trauma emergencies

A 'Medical' emergency is one brought about by a patient's illness or existing medical problems. 'Trauma' is force that has caused an injury to the patient.

Whenever 'trauma' is involved we attempt to learn about the 'Mechanism of Injury' (what happened to cause the injury). This helps us form a 'worst case scenario' of what could be wrong, and helps us to treat the patient in an aggressive manner. We should be concerned that a significant force could have caused injury to the spine (the neck and back). This complication could result in paralysis if we are not careful when examining and moving the patient. (The patient's body should be kept 'in-line', being careful not to twist or bend them.) In suspected spinal injury the rescuer holds the patient's head still and does not let go unless relieved by other rescuers. For patients with suspected spinal trauma you will need several trained rescuers to safely move and transport the patient. Your best treatment is stabilization of the neck with your hands, keeping the patient's body immobile, and waiting for the arrival of professional rescuers. Gather a medical history and do a quick body check while waiting.

The 60 Second or 'Initial' Exam

During your initial patient exam, along with insuring the A, B, C's, you will simultaneously check (visualize) the patient for obvious signs of injury such as serious bleeding, deformity of extremities, bruising, and unusual 'skin signs' (color, temperature, and moisture). Within the first minute you should also determine the patient's 'Chief Complaint', the main thing the patient complains of. Of course if a life-threatening condition is encountered your 60 Second Exam will pause as you act to handle that situation. (The 60 Second Exam will take no more than a minute only if no serious conditions requiring your action are discovered).

Skin signs:

• *Pale*: may indicate 'shock' (lack of 'perfusion': blood flow to the vital organs) or low blood pressure. This patient may be confused or dizzy.

• *Bluish*: (Cyanotic) usually indicates lack of oxygen. This patient is often short of breath, usually with either rapid shallow breathing or slow, insufficient breathing. You will often need to assist this person's breathing, and consider 'shock position.'

• *Flushed*: (red) may indicate heat stroke, or elevated blood pressure.

• *Yellowish*: (Jaundice) may indicate hepatitis (liver infection). May be infectious.

• *Cool*: may indicate 'shock,' low blood pressure, or a sign of exposure to cold.

• *Hot*: may indicate heat stroke or infection.

• *Sweaty*: may be a sign of 'shock,' low blood pressure, or heat distress. Medical conditions such as 'heart attack' may cause sweaty skin.

Shock:

(Insufficient 'oxygenated' blood flow to the vital organs)

Shock is often present in serious illnesses or injuries. The patient's 'skin signs' are your most obvious indicator of shock. If pale, cool, and moist or sweaty skin is seen, or if 'fainting' seems likely, you should treat the patient for shock. 'Shock Position' is the placing of your patient on their back with their legs raised up about 18". This may increase blood flow to the brain and other vital organs by raising the patient's blood pressure. •Warning: If the patient seems to have serious trouble breathing, especially if you hear the sound of fluid in the lungs as they breathe, do not lay them down (this could cause increased trouble in breathing). If your patient has signs of a 'stroke' (one-sided paralysis, one-sided facial drooping, slurred speech) do not lay them down (this could raise their blood pressure making the stroke worse).

Serious bleeding:

(Always use latex type gloves to avoid contact with blood)

'Arterial bleeding' may be 'spurting' type bleeding and can be life threatening if not stopped.

Direct pressure at the injury site using a clean cloth or sterile dressing is the best way to stop bleeding. Do not release the pressure until the patient is turned over to a medical professional.

The Complete Body Check:
(The Head-to-toe exam)

Beginning at the patient's head you will 'visualize' for signs of injury, then 'palpate' (feel) each area for signs of pain, swelling, and deformity. If a life-threatening problem is encountered you should first take care of that problem, then return to your complete body check if possible. You may need to cut away clothing to visualize the body for trauma. *(Remember that in most areas your ALS help is not far away. As a 'first-aid' provider you are not expected to do all the things the professional rescuers might do, but you should be able to assess the patient for life-threatening problems and treat them if you can)*

Head: Look for blood or clear drainage (may be Cerebral Spinal Fluid, CSF) from the ears and nose; this could indicate a skull fracture. Check the pupils, they should be equal in size and equally reactive to light. Widely dilated pupils may indicate lack of oxygen to the brain. Small, 'pinpoint' pupils may indicate the use of narcotics. One widely dilated pupil may indicate an injury to one part of the brain. Look in the mouth for injury, broken teeth, or other airway obstructions. Check the skull and face for injury, pain, and deformity.

Neck: Check for a 'medic alert' necklace that may tell you of the person's medical history.

Chest: Starting at the collar bones (clavicles) visualize for signs of injury; then palpate (feel) for signs of injury. Visualize and palpate the ribs.

Abdomen: Visualize for signs of injury, then begin to 'gently' palpate each 'quadrant' of the abdomen (the 'umbilicus' or belly button is the dividing line for the four quadrants, imagine a line vertically and horizontally through the umbilicus). You are checking for pain, distention, rigidity, and unusual masses.

Pelvis: Visualize for signs of injury then palpate, squeezing the pelvis at the sides then pushing at the pubic bone. You are checking for pain, instability, and deformities.

Legs: Visualize then palpate each leg for signs of injury. A fracture of the thigh bone (femur) could result in serious bleeding. Swelling at the thigh may indicate bleeding inside. Check the toes for movement (have the person gently wiggle their toes), and check for normal sensation by touching the feet and asking the patient if they feel your touch and if it feels normal to them. Check 'bilaterally' (both sides) and compare.

Arms: Visualize then palpate each arm for signs of injury. Check the wrists for medic alert bracelets and check the hands for movement and sensation, compare each side.

Back: You can slide your hand under the small of the back to check for possible hidden bleeding. If you suspect spinal injury do not turn your patient to check the back.

•You may need to remove clothing to visualize the body for signs of injury. Rather than risking movement that may cause further injury, it may be best to cut away the clothing with rescue scissors. Obviously your good judgement should guide you as to when such an exam is useful or necessary. Most often the medical professionals responding to your 9-1-1 call are not far away, and often it is best to allow 'them' to conduct the detailed body check. Always try to maintain your patient's privacy and dignity if you must remove clothing.

Vital signs:

(Breathing rate, pulse rate, blood pressure)
These measurements, along with skin signs and a check of the patient's pupil response (whether the pupils close down, 'constrict', when exposed to light; and whether the pupils are equal in size) will often give you an indication of the seriousness of the person's condition. If the pupils stay large (dilated) and don't react or react sluggishly to light, this can indicate bleeding in the brain, requiring prompt medical intervention at a hospital.

Breathing: Should be about 12 breaths a minute and without any unusual sounds such as wheezing or fluid sounds. The breath sounds should be equal on each side if you listen with a stethoscope. •Labored breathing, or lack of significant air flow with each breath, especially if accompanied by bluish colored skin ('cyanosis' which indicates lack of oxygen), require you to provide 'rescue breathing' for the patient.

Pulse: Should be approximately 80 beats per minute. Less than 60 a minute or more than 100 per minute are considered abnormal. If you feel 'skipped' beats, an irregular pulse, this may indicate an unusual or dangerous heart rhythm.

Blood pressure: If you are trained in the use of the 'sphygmomanometer' or blood pressure cuff, you should obtain a blood pressure 'after' your initial assessment and after your complete body check. Blood pressures below 90 'systolic' (the top number), or greater than 140 'systolic,' are generally considered abnormal. A patient with a low blood pressure should be placed in shock position. A patient with a high blood pressure should be kept sitting up.
•Any time a patient is 'unconscious' you should lay them down on their side or in shock position.

Critical Emergencies:

Critical emergencies are those illnesses, injuries or situations in which some prompt and appropriate intervention is necessary to prevent further complications or additional problems.

You will focus on these situations in which your actions can truly have a positive effect. Other first aid, although sometimes helpful, may be better delayed until the arrival of professional rescuers. Always remember that the actions you take may have possible negative side effects or risks to the patient. When appropriate act! But know when it is wiser to wait.

Consider a person with an obviously fractured leg. Let's say there is no other injury and no bleeding. You 'could' gather the appropriate equipment to place the injured leg in a splint. Even if you have the correct equipment available and are familiar with splinting is it wise to splint the leg? Probably not. It is probably better to simply call 9-1-1, keep the patient calm, gather any medical history, and keep them from moving the injured part. Since there is no life-threatening situation here, and because the professional rescuers will have the right equipment, proper manpower, and more expertise, you are better to delay this care to avoid possible complications during your treatment of this patient.

Wounds and bleeding: A small wound can be cleaned with soap and water. Larger wounds that will probably require stitching to repair are best simply covered with a moist dressing. (Sterile 'saline' solution is preferred, but wetting the dressing with plain water is acceptable).

A moist dressing will help preserve the tissue at the site and protect the wound from further contamination. 'Closing' a large laceration with 'butterfly bandages' should be done before covering the wound. You do not need to spend much time cleansing a large wound since it must be completely irrigated and cleaned at the hospital. As always 'direct pressure' is the most helpful technique to control serious bleeding. Once a bleeding wound is covered do not remove the dressing. If it soaks through simply put a fresh dressing 'on top' of the old one, and apply more pressure continuously. A 'tourniquet' (that stops all blood flow to an extremity) is almost never used by professional rescuers. In the vast majority of cases, even with amputations, you should be able to control serious bleeding with firm direct pressure at the site of the bleeding. Of course if you cannot control bleeding with direct pressure, quickly apply a tourniquet as close to the injury as possible. Internal bleeding is a surgical emergency requiring rapid transport.

Amputations: Stop bleeding with direct pressure. Place any amputated part in a sealed plastic bag if available, then place the bag on ice to keep it 'cool', not frozen, and bring it to the hospital with the patient.

Fractures and dislocations: We should always consider a painful, swollen area as a possible fracture site. If obvious deformity is present, or if bone ends are visible the fracture may be obvious. Our best intervention is making sure the effected part remains immobile. If a bone end is protruding, we should cover it with a moist dressing. Usually splinting in the field by first-aiders should be avoided, unless medical care is unable to respond (as in a disaster situation). If you must move the patient, then you should splint possible fractures first.

If splinting is to be done you should check the pulse, movement, and sensation (PMS) in the affected extremity before and after splinting. Your splint should immobilize the joint 'above and below' the fracture site, and the splint should be padded and 'firmly' in place to avoid movement of the splinted part. *If there is some loss of pulse, movement, or sensation after applying the splint, do not readjust the splint or the fractured part, just inform rescuers when they arrive that there was a change after splinting.*

Eye injuries: Although not usually a life-threatening emergency, an injury to the eye must be carefully treated to avoid additional damage.

Key points:
        • Do not put pressure on the eyeball. Loss of the fluid inside the eye can lead to blindness
        • An injured eye should be covered with a moist dressing. Cover only the affected eye, and, if there may be an impaled object in the eye, try to have the patient look at a fixed object to keep the eyes as still as possible. *(Covering both eyes causes 'both' eyes to move randomly and toward any sounds, which is not advised).*

The covering of only the affected eye or both eyes is an area of disagreement in first-aid textbooks and EMS delivery systems; we will consider covering only the injured eye here.

Heat Stroke: 'Heat Stroke' is the life-threatening heat emergency. Other conditions such as heat exhaustion or heat cramps may cause nausea, dizziness, and cramping, but are usually corrected by removing the person from the hot environment, removing clothing, and giving sips of water or 'Gatorade' type drinks. In Heat Stroke the patient will have developed a serious internal temperature causing confusion, flushed skin, or even unconsciousness. You must rapidly cool this patient by getting them out of the hot environment, removing their clothing, and rapidly cooling their body with wet towels and cold packs in the armpits and groin. (These areas have large arteries near the surface that can help cool the body). The head should also be wetted with water to aid in cooling.

Since these patients are usually unconscious or confused, do not give sips of water. This is true of 'any' patient who is confused (Altered Level of Consciousness, ALOC).

Cold Emergencies: As first aiders we do not want to re-warm areas of frostbite (frostbite means the part is frozen; usually pale, and numb). Do not let the patient walk or use frostbit areas. Rapid transport to the hospital while keeping the patient warm and removing wet clothing is our best action. The 'Hypothermic' patient has been exposed to cold for a prolonged period and has a lowered body temperature. The main sign is confusion and shivering. The same treatment of removing wet clothes, covering them with blankets, placing them in a heated environment, and rapid transport for medical care is our best treatment.

Burns: The modern terms for first, second, and third degree burns are 'Partial Thickness' and 'Full Thickness' burns. The thickness refers to the layers of the skin, with a third degree burn effecting the 'full thickness', or all layers, of the skin. Partial thickness burns are anything from reddening (sunburn), to blisters. Third degree burns can be obvious such as 'charred' skin, but may also be present in burned skin showing severe blistering. We are not always sure what 'type' of burn the patient has, but our treatment is the same for all burns.

Cool all burns with water (use cool tap or cool hose water). This is the first step, to stop the burning process. (If dry a chemical is on the skin, brush it off before applying water).
- *Cover the burned area with a clean dry dressing.*
- *Do not apply 'any' ointments! *See note*

Electrical burns may involve an entrance and an exit wound, the exit is often at the feet but may be any place where the patient became 'grounded' when the electricity left the body.

*Note: If you know the ointment you have is water-based, designed specifically for treating burns, and easily washed off, you could use it; such ointments sometimes soothe the pain. Many ointments however are oil-based and must be scrubbed off with a brush at the hospital!

A good rule is to use only water to cool the burn and no ointments. (You may also continue to pour water over the dressing covering the burn to help relieve pain, but wet dressings on burns for long periods should be avoided since this could damage skin, and in large burned areas, could cause hypothermia).

Breathing emergencies: This is one of the most potentially life-threatening problems. As with any emergency you should have 9-1-1 resources on the way. Someone with trouble breathing may have an airway obstruction. Your determination of 'what happened' will help you decide if airway obstruction maneuvers (abdominal thrusts/Heimlich maneuver) are appropriate. An airway obstruction may also be caused by swelling (from trauma, toxic exposure, or allergic reaction) in this case the only treatment is medications and/or special airway devices at the hospital or with the Paramedics. You can attempt to 'assist' the patient's breathing to force air past this type of 'anatomical' obstruction, while transporting or awaiting Paramedics.

'Congestive Heart Failure' (CHF) is a heart condition in which blood pressure can cause fluid to 'back up' into the lungs. This build-up of fluid will cause increasing shortness of breath (SOB), and can lead to the patient 'drowning' in their own fluids. In the beginning stages of CHF, you may hear a 'crackling' sound (Rales) when listening at the chest with a stethoscope. As the condition worsens the sound may become a 'bubbling' type of wet sound with each breath.

Do not lay these patients down unless they become unconscious. Assist their breathing and give oxygen if available until Paramedics arrive.

Other conditions such as Asthma, Emphysema, Bronchitis, Pneumonia, etc. may cause shortness of breath, wheezing, coughing, and phlegm production. Keep patients with trouble breathing sitting up, as long as they are conscious, and assist their breathing if it is less than 12 breaths a minute or if you feel they are not moving a normal volume of air with each breath, regardless of how fast these breaths might be. *Any 'noisy' breathing is a sign of serious trouble.*

Chest pain & Heart Attacks: The warning signs of 'Heart Attack' are:

- Chest pain or 'pressure' (even the feeling of gas or indigestion)
- Pale, cool, moist skin (signs of shock)
- Nausea and/or vomiting
- Pain going to the left arm, or jaw (may be a 'toothache' type complaint)
- Irregular (skipped) heart beats
- Slow pulse (Bradycardia) less than 60/min.

Obviously many other conditions may have some of these signs and symptoms, but we should treat our patients as if they have the 'worst' condition we can think of. You are always safer to consider the worst-case scenario, which keeps you from under-treating your patient.

- *Place the patient on their back, feet raised (shock position)*
- *Keep them calm*
- *Give oxygen if available (nasal cannula at 6 liters)*
- *Avoid giving any water or fluids (this is always our general rule, to help avoid vomiting)*
- *Gather a medical history, take vital signs, and keep the scene calm and quiet*

AED: In case the patient having a heart attack goes into cardiac arrest (no breathing, no pulse) you need to insure that you have a 'defibrillator' on the way! Most fire departments have equipped their fire engines with 'Automatic' defibrillators with which the firefighters can deliver a defibrillation shock. The 'fire engine' may arrive before the Paramedics; they have trained firefighter EMT rescuers, oxygen, first aid equipment, and a defibrillator. Always call 9-1-1 immediately for breathing of heart related complaints!

A 'heart attack' means death of heart tissue (Myocardial Infarction, M.I.). These can be minor, with little damage to the heart, or large, causing cardiac arrest and death.

Chest and Head injuries: Chest injuries, including broken ribs, will often cause pain as the patient inhales. Keep the patient calm and limit their movement. Assist their breathing if it is not adequate. There is no other good first aid treatment for broken ribs. All chest injuries require prompt medical care.

Head injuries may involve injury to the neck and spine, may create bleeding into the airway, and may involve damage to the brain. Our first concern is to maintain adequate breathing, while protecting the neck from movement. If spinal injury is suspected the patient is kept lying down and care is taken not to bend or twist the patient's body.

• If a stroke is suspected the patient should be kept sitting, if conscious.

Normally if you cannot ventilate the patient in the position they are found you must use the 'Head-tilt/Chin-lift to open the airway. With a suspected head injury, you must first attempt the 'Modified jaw thrust' (lifting the bottom jaw only with your fingers, with your thumbs on the patient's cheek bones). If this method fails to open the airway you can then use the Head-tilt/Chin-lift, slightly tilting at first, progressing until you are able to ventilate.

• The most obvious signs of head injury are 'blown pupils' (widely dilated and non-reactive). If both pupils are dilated we suspect a severe lack of oxygen to the entire brain, as would be expected in a cardiac arrest patient. If only one pupil is 'blown' we suspect an injury to a specific portion of one side of the brain, as in a traumatic blow to the head, or stroke. Rapid transport to the hospital while maintaining the airway is most important.

Abdominal injury: This may present as pain, distention, rigidity, or bruising in the abdominal quadrants. The concern is that internal bleeding may be occurring requiring surgery. Generally, 'shock position' is indicated where internal bleeding may be occurring.

You may also consider drawing the patient's knees toward the chest, this may relieve some pain by taking tension off the abdominal muscles.

Rapid transport to the hospital with oxygen if available. (All serious patients should have oxygen if available).

Stroke: *Cerebral Vascular Accident or CVA* is a stroke. Some new texts are referring to stroke as 'Brain Attack'. A stroke is a brain injury from either bleeding from or blockage of a vessel. Whatever the cause the result is a lack of oxygen to a portion of the brain.

Signs:
- One-sided paralysis or weakness, and/or altered level of consciousness/confusion
- Facial drooping on one side
- Slurred speech or the inability to speak
- Severe headache

Stroke is often brought about by high blood pressure (Hypertension). A patient is considered 'hypertensive' if their blood pressure is greater than 140 systolic (top number), or greater than 90 diastolic (the bottom number). If 'either' or both number is above these maximum limits your patient is at risk.

Keep the patient with suspected stroke in a sitting position, to avoid extra blood pressure to the brain, which may increase the stroke damage.

Diabetic emergencies: A diabetic emergency is rarely life threatening, and is best handled by 9-1-1 responders. The patient in a diabetic emergency is most often confused, and sometimes combative.

• A diabetic has a medical condition in which the body's normal balance of sugar is disrupted. The pancreas produces 'insulin' which is needed to regulate sugar to the cells. 'Hypoglycemia' or Insulin Shock is a low sugar condition, which may occur suddenly if the patient has not eaten properly or has been working strenuously. Giving this patient sugar, if they are alert

enough to drink a drink with sugar added, will temporarily improve their condition. 'Hyperglycemia' or Diabetic Coma is an elevated sugar condition often taking several days to develop. This is more serious than Hypoglycemia and your patient will most often be unconscious.

You can give sips of a sugary drink to the confused diabetic, if you are sure they are diabetic, and if they are able to hold and drink the drink by themselves.

<u>Poisoning and overdose</u>: This is another situation in which we have no safe and effective first-aid intervention. Call 9-1-1, treat for shock if present, assist breathing if needed, do not induce vomiting, and place the patient in 'recovery' position (on their side) if they have an altered level of consciousness.

• Gather any medications or substances (if safe to handle) if they have been poisoned or have overdosed. These should be sent to the hospital with the patient.

<u>Seizure</u>: Also known as a 'convulsion,' these patients often experience violent full body shaking, during a period of unconsciousness. Seizures are often associated with past brain injury, some medication overdoses, or brain tumors, although some seizure disorders have no known cause. If the patient has a past history of seizures, they are probably on daily medication to help control them. Most seizures will last less than a minute and are often followed by a period of confusion or sleepiness (the 'Post Ictal' state).

• Never put anything in the patient's mouth. They 'may' bite their tongue but this will probably have already happened as the

seizure began, and is usually minor. The seizing patient cannot 'swallow' their tongue.

• Move objects out of the way during a seizure. The patient may strike themselves against objects and become injured.

• Since the Post Ictal state is normal, do not try to quickly arouse the patient after the seizure. As long as they are breathing you can place them in recovery position (on their side) and await the Paramedics.

• Oxygen is helpful if you have it available, and if the confused patient will tolerate it.

Allergic reaction: Also known as 'Anaphylactic shock' in severe cases.

      <u>Signs</u>: Hives, itching, swelling, difficulty breathing.

Rapid transport to the hospital with oxygen (or assist breathing if needed)

Paramedics carry medications useful in reversing the symptoms

Bites and stings: Animal bites usually require simple washing with soap and water and follow up with a doctor to treat possible infection and/or damage to nerves, vessels, tendons, muscle, and bone; basically, 'wound care'. Insect stings or bites have a greater potential for dangerous allergic reactions. Most care for insect bites involves ointments to reduce itching, or swelling, but infection and disease transmission is a concern with any insect bite or sting. Reptiles such as poisonous snakes present a possible life threat, although most people bitten by poisonous snakes in the United States do survive. There is no effective first aid. Treatment for rattlesnake bites involves the in-hospital administration of an anti-venin. Some texts will talk of 'constricting bands' (which is not a tourniquet), and immobilizing the affected part.

Keep the patient calm, do not let them walk, and get them to the hospital.

Never cut or suck the wound. This does not remove venom and risks infection at the site.

Do not attempt to catch the snake. The anti-venin is a made for any type of rattlesnake, so it won't necessarily matter to the hospital which type bit the patient.

Childbirth: Your main concern after a normal delivery is in keeping the baby warm. Of course rescue breathing and/or CPR would be started if necessary. You should wait for professional rescuers to arrive and let them cut the umbilical cord; there is no hurry to cut the cord. Other complications of childbirth are beyond the scope of the first aider and can be studied in EMT/Paramedic textbooks.

If the mother shows signs of shock or excess bleeding place her in shock position and give oxygen if available. Allow the mother to breast-feed the baby; this helps the uterus contract to prevent excess bleeding.

Other concerns: Your calm action and common sense will help you handle other unusual situations that you may come upon. Remember that help is usually not far away, and the basic principles taught to you here should help you to decide on the most appropriate course of action in difficult situations. Doing the best you can while using good judgement, and always trying to do what is best for the patient is all that can be expected of you.

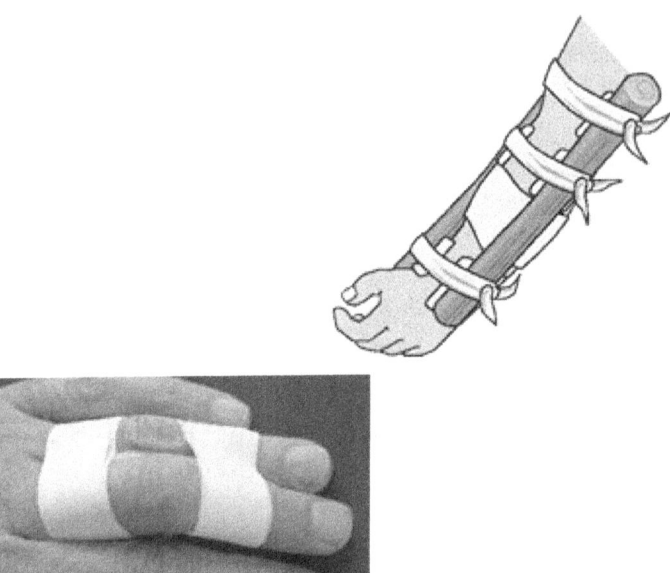

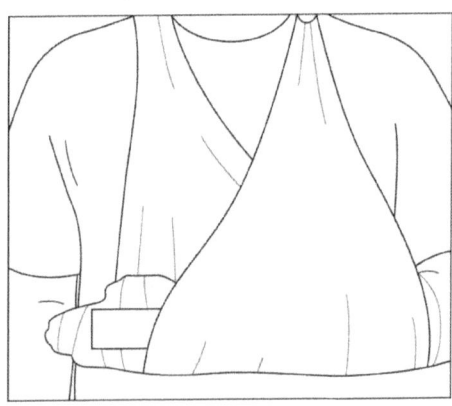

Disaster Preparedness

<u>Disaster</u>: A situation which overwhelms available resources

Common sense and the ability to organize

A 'disaster' can take many shapes. From a computer system out of service at a bank, to an earthquake, the meaning of disaster can vary. For our purposes we most often think of 'natural disasters' related to acts of nature, and this is a good model to develop preparedness plans.

The main thing to remember is that during a 'disaster' your normal way of handling emergencies will change. Calling 9-1-1 will get you a recording, if the phone system is working. Emergency agencies such as police, fire, and Paramedics will be unavailable! Many structures may be damaged, including police, fire stations, and hospitals. A mobilization of the National Guard and other relief agencies will occur but will take time. Most disaster planners talk of three days 'on your own'.

Preparedness. Being prepared takes planning. If you plan to be self-sufficient for three days or more, you must think it out carefully. Utilities may be out; no gas for cooking or heating, no water for drinking or to make the toilets function, no electricity for lights or appliances, no phones, no television or radio, no access to banks or auto tellers! Stores will be closed; martial law may be ordered to prevent looting which may keep you from traveling at certain times. Roads will be damaged, highways impassable, fires may be sweeping though vast areas, the water systems damaged, hospitals, firefighters, police, EMT's and Paramedics overwhelmed.

During a major earthquake in California for example, state planners 'expect' *thousands* dead. The disruption in services will be vast, the prospect of hundreds of others dying days later from moderate injuries is real, the spread of disease is expected, and the recovery of normal 'services' will take many months! This same scenario could exist for other disasters such as floods, tornadoes, severe weather, tsunamis, even hazardous materials incidents. There is a potential risk of some sort of disaster striking you and your family no matter who you are or where you live.

<u>Key points</u>:

• Have significant 'cash' available in 'small bills'

• Develop a family meeting plan if separated

• Family members have the phone number of an 'out of state' contact person

• Have water and food available to last 'at least' three days

• Prepare a 'backpack' with essentials: money, medications, car/house keys, glasses/contacts, hearing aids, etc.

Think it out! Proper planning could make it less of a disaster for you

The entire family should be involved in planning. Everyone needs to know' The plan'.

Cash:

Banks may not be available for some time. You may find some stores open or items for sale by individuals. Getting change for large bills may be difficult. If you're forced to buy needed items they will be expensive.

The meeting place:

Every family member should know the family meeting place. It can be your home, a park, a school, a church. Remember that some large areas such as parks, schoolyards, and churches, may become community gathering places (and may be mini disasters themselves due to crowds). Have a secondary or even a third potential meeting place planned in case your first choice is not available for some reason.

Out-of-state contact:

When local phone systems go out you may not be able to connect to nearby areas, since these areas may depend on telephone 'wires' to work. You may be able to call out of state since those systems often rely on wireless signals. Family members can call this out of state contact and use them as a message relay to tell each other that you are O.K., where you are, and where and when you will meet.

Water and food:

Water comes first. You can survive weeks without food, but only days without water. Bottled water sufficient for several days should be stored and 'rotated' with fresh water every six months. (You should plan at least 1 gallon of water per day for 'every' family member). Food should be 'ready to eat' such as: granola, canned tuna, canned fruits, peanut butter/crackers, beef jerky, and powdered drink mixes. All foods are safest when rotated about every six months (mark each container with the date stored and the date to rotate). Don't forget to store a can opener 'with' the canned food.

The 'backpack':
You may need to leave your house quickly. If you don't have the ability to gather supplies at least your emergency backpack can be easily taken with you. In it you should have some essentials; cash, vital medications, extra set of keys, glasses/contacts (contact storing and cleaning equipment), and other items you would have a hard time living without. The backpack should have 'space blankets' for emergency shelter; an old but sturdy pair of shoes in case you have to rush out bare-footed, leather gloves for moving debris, flashlights and extra batteries, and some water and food. The items in your pack may be the only items you will have if a fire occurs or severe structural damage keeps you from reentering your home.

First Aid supplies:
Simple first aid supplies, mostly for dealing with cuts, should be of sufficient quantity for several people for several days. You can make your own items by taking a clean white sheet and cutting it into a dozen or more 4" wide strips about 6' long, and roll them (for 'bandage'

material). Cut dozens of 6x6" 'squares' to use as 'dressing' materials. Store these items in zip-lock type storage bags along with some 'Bactine' type spray antiseptic and an anti-bacterial ointment. Butterfly bandages are useful in closing large lacerations. Rescue scissors should be available to cut bandage material, and/or cut away clothing. Tweezers are useful as well. You don't need to spend a fortune on first aid supplies, keep it simple, and have more dressing and bandage material than you think you need! If you include medications, check expiration dates frequently.

Other supplies:
Sunscreen, lip balm, radio and extra batteries, clothes (hat, thermal underwear, jacket, rain poncho, blankets/sleeping bags, tent, eating utensils, and liquid detergent; also toilet paper, plastic garbage bags and plastic bucket (for sanitation uses), chlorine bleach 'plain' not scented (8 drops per gallon to disinfect water), moistened 'towelettes', sturdy utility knife, long burning candles, waterproof matches, towels, toothpaste/tooth brushes, paper towels, shampoo, tools (large crescent wrench, shovel, hammer/nails, crowbar, rope, plastic sheeting roll, gloves, dust masks) careful planning will help you develop 'your' list of needs.

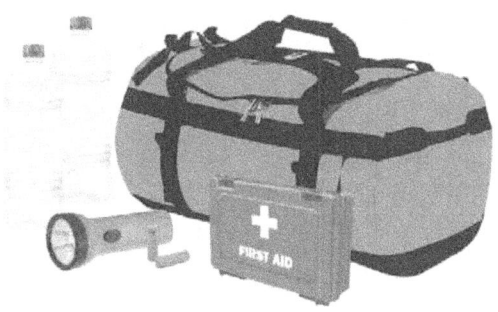

Disaster Preparedness Checklist

Gather disaster items NOW. Make sure your family is aware of your disaster plans, the location of emergency supplies (backpack), and discuss your family response to a disaster at least once a year.

☐ 'Cash' available in 'small bills' sufficient for 'at least' one week.

☐ Develop a family meeting plan if separated, to include a secondary meeting place.

☐ Family members have the phone number of an 'out of state' contact person.

☐ Have water and food available to last 'at least' one week.

☐ Prepare a 'backpack' with essentials: first aid supplies, money, medications, car/house keys, glasses/contacts, hearing aids, etc.

☐ Family members know how to shut off the gas.

☐ Family members know where the fire extinguishers are.

☐ Family members know where the emergency backpack is.

☐ The disaster plan has been discussed with all family members.

Think it out! Proper planning could make it less of a disaster for you.

The entire family should be involved in planning.

Everyone needs to know' The plan'

Self-Defense

#1 Get away if you can! But, if you have to fight, make sure you win!

Your life is at stake. You must become focused, you must disable the attacker quickly and get away. You may not get a second chance!

Self-Defense is a simple concept. Your goal is to protect yourself from attack and or injury. This WILL involve hurting your attacker if you are forced to confront them directly.

The most important first step in self-defense is to 'avoid' a potentially dangerous situation. Remember common sense principles such as avoiding being alone, especially at night, and staying out of dark or remote areas, areas where someone could hide, or areas known for high crime rates.

The problem is that there are times when you cannot avoid such situations; it is your ability to recognize the 'potential' danger, remain alert, and be prepared to take appropriate action that makes you better able to respond quickly to protect yourself.

Confrontation. If you find yourself suddenly confronted by an individual or group of potential attackers you must act quickly, your response should be pre-planned and occur suddenly and with determination. A constant goal is to keep a significant distance between you and the attacker. Getting away is always your best option. To simply run toward other people or into a business is one of the best first actions. If you are in a remote location and have a personal protection device (pepper spray or other weapon) consider using it and then escaping. You can avoid using a defensive weapon on an innocent person by yelling loudly "I have a weapon, stay back." If the person continues to advance and you truly feel your life is in danger you have every right to defend yourself, this includes the use of deadly force.

• If attacked fight back HARD and don't give up

• If grabbed, drop quickly to the ground to break away

• Use your elbows and knees to deliver sharp, rapid blows

• Strike the face, neck, groin with rapid, forceful strikes

• You 'are' trying to cause injury, including broken bones

• When you think you have caused injury strike again to disable your attacker, allowing you to flee

Important points:
• Carry pepper spray or other weapons, know how to use the device, and have it 'in your hand' when in a potentially dangerous area. Prepare to use it!

• Be aware of people around you, stay away from vans or vehicles with a person(s) in them or parked next to your car. Enter on the passenger side if a potential threat exists on the driver's side.

• Pay special attention when unlocking your vehicle and getting in. Pay attention for people who may come up behind you. Get in your car quickly and lock the door first.

• Pre-plan your actions. If a situation occurs, you must act instinctively!

• If attacked be prepared to be injured. Don't give up when hurt! Assume that you are likely to be killed if your attacker wins. Fight for your life!

• Practice punching and kicking. Workout videos such as Tae-Bo are excellent.

Protecting yourself and your loved ones during an attack takes special preparation, both physical and mental. Do not underestimate an attacker's determination! You must be equally determined to keep yourself safe and defeat the attacker. Be ruthless; make sure you damage them severely! Don't hold back, and persist until you are safe!

Closing thoughts:

There are many other items to consider when thinking of 'preparedness' in general. It is not only your ability to quickly recognize and appropriately treat those injured or ill, and not only your ability to 'survive' a serious disruption in your normal life, as in a disaster, but perhaps most importantly your ability to organize and direct others.

An emergency situation will test your ability to remain thoughtful and organized in the face of severe stress. It is this quality which makes the professional rescuer 'seem' so calm and in control during an emergency. It is 10% practice and exposure to these situations, and 90% 'preparedness'. The professional rescuer knows what to do, and that makes their actions quick, efficient, and appropriate.

Your ability to direct others to call for help, or to control and organize bystanders while providing appropriate first care, is what makes you a 'rescuer'. Your ability to 'focus' is what can keep you safe.

It is the goal of this book to better prepare you to act. Above all it is 'action' that counts. Being able to not only 'do something', but to do the 'right' thing. Of course no training program and no book can discuss 'every' situation that may occur, it is your common sense along with a basic understanding of the principles we have discussed that will allow you to handle a situation you had never thought of before.

Learn as much as you can, review this material frequently, certify in CPR and First Aid annually, learn and practice self-defense techniques, and be 'prepared'.

Lance Hodge

There is much 'free' literature available from emergency agencies such as the American Red Cross, the American Heart Association, FEMA (the Federal Emergency Management Agency), the Governor's Office of Emergency Services, local fire departments, your City, and even the front of most phone books are full of valuable information on first aid and preparedness.

General Guidelines for CPR and Choking

<u>CPR/CHOKING Techniques</u>

USE GLOVES, EYE PROTECTION, AND MOUTH BARRIER DEVICE
OR BVM TO AVOID CONTACT WITH BODY FLUIDS

CHECK RESPONSIVENESS: Shout! "Are you OK?"
then tap shoulder firmly!
IF UNRESPONSIVE: Call 9-1-1
RAPID DEFIBRILLATION IS THE KEY TO SURVIVAL IN CARDIAC ARREST!

A-B-C's (New: C-A-B) Compressions-Airway-Breaths

*Open airway with Head tilt/chin lift (if no trauma)
'Observe' for signs of life/breathing: **Look, Listen, Feel while checking carotid PULSE for 5 seconds.**

C- If no signs of movement, breathing, or pulse, start CPR chest Compressions (30) see Chest Compressions below

A-B Open the Airway and give (two) slow full Breaths (stop breath when chest rises)

If unable to get breath in, re-tilt head and try again 'several times', if still unable to get breath in, go to: *Choking/Airway Obstruction: Unconscious, now.*

NOTE: Infants & Children: Give CPR if pulse is less than 60/min. with signs of poor perfusion (blue, limp, no response)

(Lay rescuers are taught to check for signs of normal breathing and/or movement, and not to check the pulse)

(Infant: Check 'brachial' pulse in upper arm for (5) seconds) If pulse is present, see Rescue Breathing

AED – Use AED/defibrillator if available, can be used on adults, children, and infants (refer to the specific AED) attach AED only if no breathing/movement/pulse

The AED is simple, open lid or push button to turn on, follow voice directions and pictures on patches, attach patches to chest, do not touch the person when delivering a shock!

The 'Good Samaritan Law' (for non-professional rescuers) protects you from liability when helping with 'medical' procedures in a reasonable way and in good faith. Quickly delivering an AED shock in a cardiac arrest is THE KEY to survival! Don't delay, use an AED if available!

CHEST COMPRESSIONS

ADULT: (30:2) 30 chest compressions: 2 breaths

(Professional Rescuers two-person CPR, with E.T. tube, no pause for ventilations)

Adult depth of compressions: at least 2 inches (heel of hand between nipple line)

Adult rate: at 100-120 compressions/minute- Count: "One, and Two, and Three..." ("Stayin Alive" beat)

CHILD: (1 to Adolescent)- (30:2) 30 chest compressions (heel of one or two hands between nipple line) : 2 breaths

Child depth of chest compressions: (2 inches or 1/3 of the depth of the chest)

Child rate: at least 100-120 compressions/minute- Count: "One, and Two, and Three..."

INFANT: (Newborn to 1-year-old)- (30:2) 30 compressions (use 2 fingertips on breastbone 'just' below the nipple line): 2 breaths (Just until the chest rises)

Infant depth of chest compressions: (1 ½ inches or 1/3 of the depth of the chest)

Infant rate: at least 100-120 compressions/minute- Count: "One, and Two, and Three..."

RESCUE BREATHING

If person has a pulse but is not breathing- (use 'barrier device'; pinch nose, seal around mouth) or use BVM

ADULT: Give one breath every (5) seconds
CHILD / INFANT: Give one breath every (3) seconds

CHOKING / AIRWAY OBSTRUCTION

ADULT/CHILD: Conscious- Reach around the person, place fist of one hand; thumb inward, just above belly button.

Place your other hand on top of the first; give a quick, explosive thrusts (inward and upward).

Recheck hand position, repeat thrust.

Repeat until airway is clear or person becomes unconscious.

Pregnant or obese: Use jerky 'chest thrusts'; reach around with fist on mid-sternum, not abdominal, thrust straight inward into chest

ADULT/CHILD: If they become unresponsive while doing abdominal or chest thrusts- Lay them down. Do CPR, checking the mouth for object before each breath attempt.

After chest compressions, before attempting breaths, open airway, look for foreign object, remove it if seen.

Try several times to give breaths. (If breath goes in, give 'second' breath then go to 'C' under A-B-C's)

If unable to get breath in, continue CPR chest compressions, checking mouth for object before attempting breaths.

INFANT: *Responsive*- Do not over extend infant's neck when opening airway, support head! Sandwich infant between your hands and arms, turn infant over and give (5) firm "back blows" between shoulder blades, turn infant over and give (5) jerky/quick "chest thrusts" (two fingers on chest in same position as infant CPR) Repeat until airway is clear or infant becomes unresponsive.

INFANT: *Unresponsive*- Do CPR, checking mouth for object before each breath attempt.

After chest compressions, before attempting breaths, open airway, look for foreign object, remove it if seen.

Try several times to give breaths. (If breath goes in, give 'second' breath then go to 'C' under A-B-C's)

If unable to get breath in, continue CPR chest compressions, checking mouth before attempting breaths.

~

Note: *Much of this book is simplified, it is not realistic to expect to do advanced treatment without advanced training. Much of what the EMT does (ambulance personnel, and firefighters) is 'simple' first aid, of the sort we have discussed here. It is knowing when to sit someone up, lay them down, put them on their side, or the realization that it is only advanced medical care that will be effective, that makes up most of first aid care, even for professional rescuers.*

Note:

Always bring some reading materials along on your wilderness adventures!

Other books by Lance Hodge:

The Oracle of Chadwick County

The Writer

**Secrets of my Grandfather:
A guide to Life's Wisdom**

Poetry, Thirty-Seven Years

Simple Zen

Topics

Dexter Doubletree: Volumes 1-11

The Master Works: Art

Available at:

AMAZON.com, LanceHodge.com,

Booksamillion.com, and Barnes & Noble.

www.ingramcontent.com/pod-product-compliance
Lightning Source LLC
Chambersburg PA
CBHW060209290526
45789CB00003B/1215